PLANT-BASED WEIGHT LOSS COOKBOOK

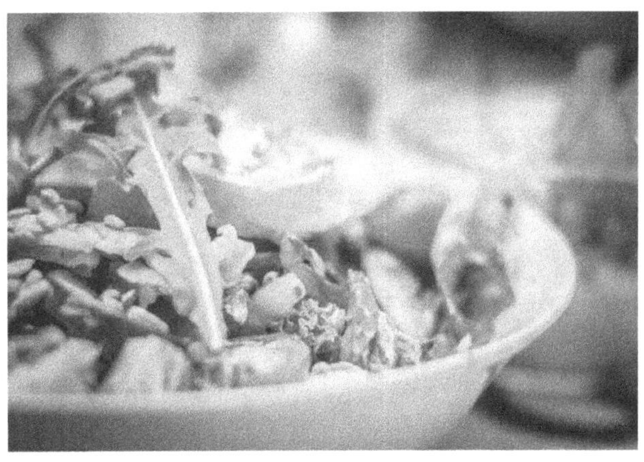

DR. JESSICA SMITH

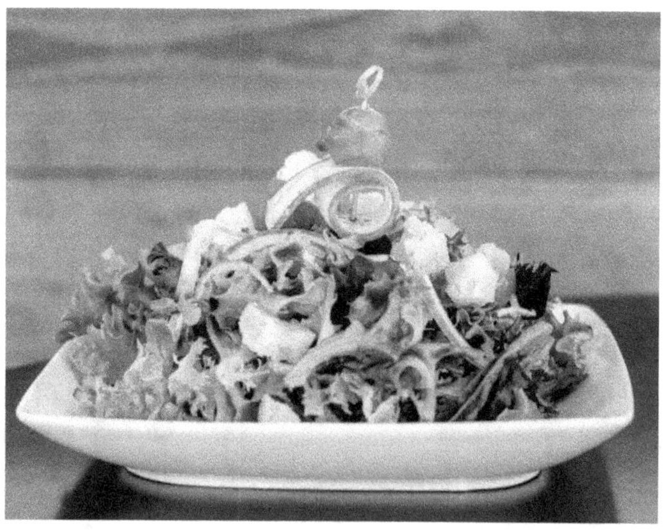

TABLE OF CONTENTS

CHAPTER ONE

How to Use this Cookbook

Research and Compile Recipes: Gather a diverse range of plant-based recipes that are not only delicious but also support weight loss goals. Include a variety of meals, snacks, and desserts to cater to different preferences and dietary needs.

Focus on Nutrient Density: Ensure that the recipes are rich in essential nutrients such as vitamins, minerals, fiber, and healthy fats. Emphasize whole, minimally processed ingredients like fruits, vegetables, whole grains, legumes, nuts, and seeds.

Create Balanced Meals: Design recipes that provide a balance of macronutrients (carbohydrates, proteins, and fats) to keep readers feeling satisfied and energized throughout the day. Incorporate a mix of complex carbohydrates, lean proteins, and healthy fats into each meal.

Control Portion Sizes: Offer guidance on portion control to help readers manage their calorie intake effectively.

Provide serving sizes for each recipe and tips on how to listen to hunger cues to prevent overeating.

Experiment with Flavor: Explore various herbs, spices, and seasoning blends to enhance the taste of plant-based dishes without relying on excessive amounts of salt, sugar, or unhealthy fats. Encourage readers to get creative in the kitchen and customize recipes to suit their taste preferences.

Include Practical Tips: Provide practical tips and tricks for meal planning, grocery shopping, food preparation, and cooking techniques to make the transition to a plant-based diet easier and more enjoyable.

Offer Substitution Options: Offer substitution options for common allergens or dietary restrictions to ensure that the recipes are inclusive and accessible to a wide range of individuals. Include alternatives for ingredients like gluten, soy, nuts, and dairy.

Provide Nutritional Information: Offer nutritional information for each recipe, including calorie count, macronutrient breakdown, and key vitamins and minerals.

This allows readers to make informed choices about their food intake and track their progress towards their weight loss goals.

Promote Sustainable Lifestyle Changes: Encourage readers to view the cookbook as a tool for long-term health and wellness rather than a quick-fix solution. Emphasize the importance of incorporating regular physical activity, staying hydrated, getting adequate sleep, and managing stress for overall well-being.

Understanding Plant Based Weight Loss

Understanding plant-based weight loss involves recognizing the power of whole, plant-derived foods in promoting healthy weight management while embracing a sustainable and compassionate dietary approach.

Unlike conventional weight loss programs that often focus on calorie restriction or specific macronutrient ratios, plant-based weight loss emphasizes the consumption of nutrient-dense fruits, vegetables, whole grains, legumes, nuts, and seeds.

At its core, plant-based weight loss relies on the principles of abundance rather than deprivation.

By filling your plate with fiber-rich foods that are low in calorie density but high in volume, you can feel satisfied while naturally reducing overall calorie intake. These foods are not only nutrient-packed but also contribute to satiety, helping to control hunger and cravings.

Moreover, plant-based diets have been linked to various health benefits beyond weight loss, including improved heart health, better blood sugar control, and reduced risk of chronic diseases such as diabetes, hypertension, and certain cancers.

This holistic approach to nutrition emphasizes the importance of nourishing the body with wholesome, minimally processed foods while minimizing or eliminating animal products and highly refined foods.

In essence, understanding plant-based weight loss involves recognizing that food is not just fuel for the body but also a powerful tool for enhancing overall health and well-being.

By prioritizing whole plant foods and adopting a more plant-centric eating pattern, individuals can achieve sustainable weight loss while reaping numerous health rewards along the way.

The principles of plant-based weight loss revolve around harnessing the nutritional power of whole, plant-derived foods to promote sustainable and effective weight management.

These principles are rooted in evidence-based research and emphasize the consumption of nutrient-dense, minimally processed plant foods while minimizing or eliminating animal products and highly refined foods.

Emphasis on Whole Foods: Plant-based weight loss prioritizes whole, unprocessed plant foods such as fruits, vegetables, whole grains, legumes, nuts, and seeds. These foods are rich in fiber, vitamins, minerals, and antioxidants, promoting satiety and overall health.

Calorie Density Awareness: Plant-based diets naturally tend to be lower in calorie density due to their high fiber and water content. By focusing on foods that are low in calorie density but high in volume, individuals can feel satisfied while consuming fewer calories, facilitating weight loss.

Balanced Macronutrients: Plant-based weight loss emphasizes the importance of consuming a balanced mix of macronutrients, including carbohydrates, proteins, and fats, to support overall health and satiety. Whole plant foods provide all essential nutrients in varying proportions, ensuring a well-rounded diet.

Mindful Eating: Practicing mindful eating techniques, such as paying attention to hunger and fullness cues, savoring each bite, and eating slowly, can help individuals develop a healthier relationship with food and prevent overeating.

Regular Physical Activity: While diet plays a crucial role in weight loss, incorporating regular physical activity is also essential for overall health and sustainable weight management. Plant-based weight loss encourages individuals to engage in regular exercise to enhance calorie expenditure and promote cardiovascular health.

By adhering to these principles, individuals can adopt a plant-based eating pattern that supports their weight loss goals while promoting long-term health and well-being.

Benefits of Plant Based Weight Loss

Plant-based weight loss offers a multitude of benefits beyond just shedding pounds, encompassing improvements in overall health, sustainability, and ethical considerations.

Weight Management: Adopting a plant-based diet can facilitate weight loss due to the naturally lower calorie density of plant foods. High fiber content and water volume in fruits, vegetables, legumes, and whole grains promote satiety while controlling calorie intake.

Heart Health: Plant-based diets have been linked to lower risk factors for heart disease, including reduced cholesterol levels, blood pressure, and inflammation. By emphasizing whole plant foods rich in fiber, antioxidants, and healthy fats, individuals can support cardiovascular health and reduce the risk of heart-related issues.

Blood Sugar Control: Plant-based diets may help improve insulin sensitivity and blood sugar control, making them beneficial for individuals with diabetes or at risk of developing the condition. Whole plant foods have a lower glycemic index, leading to more stable blood sugar levels.

Gut Health: Plant-based diets are rich in fiber, which acts as a prebiotic, nourishing beneficial gut bacteria. A healthy gut microbiome is associated with improved digestion, immune function, and mood regulation.

Reduced Cancer Risk: Certain plant foods contain phytochemicals and antioxidants that may help protect against various types of cancer. By consuming a diverse range of plant foods, individuals can support their body's natural defense mechanisms against cancer development.

Environmental Sustainability: Plant-based diets have a lower environmental footprint compared to diets rich in animal products. By reducing reliance on animal agriculture, individuals can help mitigate deforestation, water depletion, and greenhouse gas emissions associated with livestock production.

Ethical Considerations: Choosing a plant-based diet aligns with ethical considerations related to animal welfare and cruelty. By opting for plant foods over animal products, individuals can contribute to the reduction of animal suffering in factory farming practices.

In summary, plant-based weight loss offers a holistic approach to health and well-being, encompassing physical health benefits, environmental sustainability, and ethical considerations.

By adopting a plant-centric eating pattern, individuals can not only achieve their weight loss goals but also promote long-term health and support broader societal and environmental goals.

Tips for Plant Based Weight Loss

Plant-based weight loss can be both effective and sustainable with the right strategies and tips tailored to this dietary approach.

Here are some helpful tips to support your plant-based weight loss journey:

Focus on Whole Foods: Base your diet around whole, minimally processed plant foods such as fruits, vegetables, whole grains, legumes, nuts, and seeds. These foods are rich in fiber, vitamins, minerals, and antioxidants, supporting satiety and overall health.

Prioritize Fiber-Rich Foods: Fiber helps you feel full and satisfied, making it easier to control portion sizes and reduce overall calorie intake. Incorporate plenty of fiber-rich foods like fruits, vegetables, whole grains, and legumes into your meals.

Include Protein in Every Meal: Plant-based sources of protein such as beans, lentils, tofu, tempeh, edamame, quinoa, and nuts/seeds are essential for muscle repair, satiety, and metabolic function. Aim to include a source of protein in every meal to support your weight loss goals.

Mindful Eating: Pay attention to your hunger and fullness cues, and practice mindful eating. Eating slowly, savoring each bite, and focusing on the taste and texture of your food can help prevent overeating and promote enjoyment of meals.

Stay Hydrated: Drink plenty of water throughout the day. Sometimes thirst can be mistaken for hunger, leading to unnecessary snacking. Hydrating adequately can help curb cravings and support overall health.

Limit Processed Foods: Minimize consumption of processed plant-based foods like vegan junk food, vegan sweets, and heavily processed meat substitutes. These foods are often high in added sugars, unhealthy fats, and sodium, which can hinder weight loss efforts.

Plan and Prepare Meals: Take time to plan your meals and snacks in advance, and batch cook whenever possible.

Having nutritious, plant-based options readily available can prevent impulse eating and help you stay on track with your weight loss goals.

Be Patient and Persistent: Sustainable weight loss takes time and consistency. Focus on making gradual, long-term changes to your eating habits rather than seeking quick fixes. Celebrate your progress along the way and remember that every healthy choice you make contributes to your overall well-being.

By incorporating these tips into your plant-based lifestyle, you can optimize your weight loss journey while enjoying a variety of delicious, nutrient-dense foods.

Guidelines for Plant Based Weight Loss

Plant-based weight loss follows certain guidelines to ensure effective and sustainable results while maintaining overall health and well-being.

Here are some key guidelines to consider:

Eat Mostly Whole Foods: Base your diet around whole, minimally processed plant foods such as fruits, vegetables, whole grains, legumes, nuts, and seeds.

These foods are rich in fiber, vitamins, minerals, and antioxidants, supporting satiety and providing essential nutrients.

Emphasize Plant Protein: Include a variety of plant-based protein sources in your meals, such as beans, lentils, tofu, tempeh, edamame, quinoa, and nuts/seeds. Protein helps maintain muscle mass, supports metabolism, and keeps you feeling full and satisfied.

Watch Portion Sizes: While plant-based foods are generally lower in calories compared to animal products, portion control is still important for weight loss. Be mindful of portion sizes, especially with higher-calorie plant foods like nuts, seeds, and grains.

Limit Added Fats and Sugars: Be cautious with added fats and sugars, even from plant-based sources. Choose healthier fats like avocado, nuts, and seeds in moderation, and limit added sugars by opting for whole fruits over fruit juices and processed sweets.

Include Plenty of Fiber: Fiber-rich foods like fruits, vegetables, whole grains, and legumes help promote satiety, regulate blood sugar levels, and support digestive health.

Aim to include a variety of fiber sources in your diet to aid in weight loss.

Stay Hydrated: Drink plenty of water throughout the day to stay hydrated and support optimal metabolism. Sometimes thirst can be mistaken for hunger, leading to unnecessary snacking.

Be Mindful of Macronutrients: Aim for a balanced intake of macronutrients—carbohydrates, proteins, and fats. While plant-based diets naturally contain carbohydrates, focus on incorporating lean proteins and healthy fats to support overall health and weight loss goals.

Stay Active: Regular physical activity is essential for overall health and weight management. Incorporate both cardiovascular exercise and strength training into your routine to maximize calorie burning and muscle maintenance.

Listen to Your Body: Pay attention to hunger and fullness cues, and eat when you're hungry, stopping when you're satisfied. Be mindful of emotional eating triggers and find alternative ways to cope with stress or boredom.

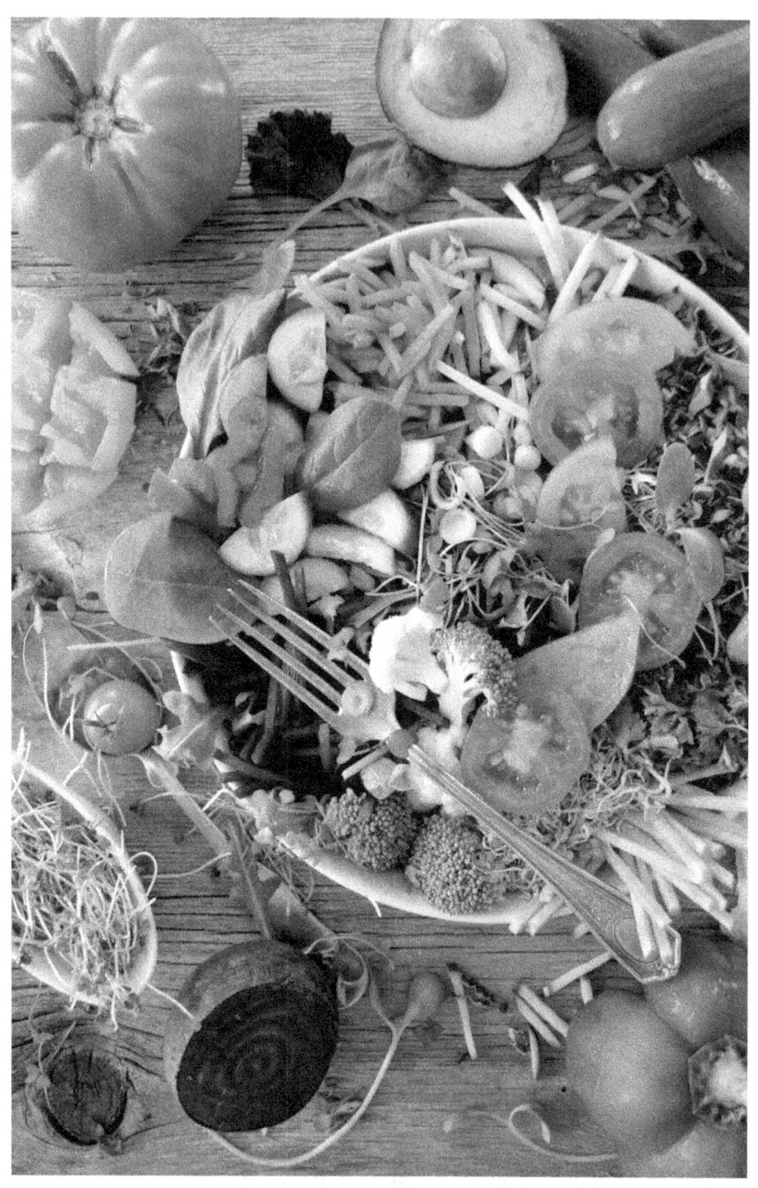

CHAPTER TWO

1. Avocado Toast with Tomato and Hemp Seeds

Ingredients:

- ➢ 2 slices of whole grain bread
- ➢ 1 ripe avocado
- ➢ 1 tomato, sliced
- ➢ 1 tablespoon hemp seeds
- ➢ Salt and pepper to taste

Instructions:

- ➢ Toast the bread slices until golden brown.
- ➢ Mash the ripe avocado and spread it evenly onto the toasted bread slices.
- ➢ Top with sliced tomatoes and sprinkle hemp seeds over the avocado.
- ➢ Season with salt and pepper to taste.
- ➢ Serve immediately.

Health Benefits:

> Avocado provides healthy fats and fiber, promoting satiety and heart health.
> Tomatoes are rich in vitamins, minerals, and antioxidants, supporting overall health and immunity.
> Hemp seeds are a good source of plant-based protein, omega-3 fatty acids, and minerals like magnesium and iron.

Preparation Time: 10 minutes

2. Berry Smoothie Bowl

Ingredients:

> 1 frozen banana
> 1 cup mixed berries (such as strawberries, blueberries, raspberries)
> 1/2 cup spinach or kale leaves
> 1/2 cup almond milk or any plant-based milk
> Toppings: sliced fruits, granola, chia seeds, shredded coconut

Instructions:

- In a blender, combine the frozen banana, mixed berries, spinach or kale, and almond milk.
- Blend until smooth and creamy, adding more almond milk if needed to reach your desired consistency.
- Pour the smoothie into a bowl.
- Top with sliced fruits, granola, chia seeds, and shredded coconut.
- Serve immediately.

Health Benefits:

- Berries are packed with antioxidants, vitamins, and fiber, supporting digestion and immune function.
- Spinach or kale adds extra fiber, vitamins, and minerals like iron and calcium.
- Chia seeds provide omega-3 fatty acids, protein, and additional fiber for satiety.

Preparation Time: 5 minutes

3. Tofu Scramble

Ingredients:

- 1/2 block firm tofu, crumbled

- ➢ 1/4 cup diced bell peppers
- ➢ 1/4 cup diced onions
- ➢ 1/2 cup spinach
- ➢ 1 tablespoon nutritional yeast
- ➢ 1/2 teaspoon turmeric powder
- ➢ Salt and pepper to taste
- ➢ Cooking oil (such as olive oil or coconut oil)

Instructions:

- ➢ Heat a skillet over medium heat and add cooking oil.
- ➢ Add diced bell peppers and onions to the skillet, and sauté until softened.
- ➢ Add crumbled tofu to the skillet, along with nutritional yeast, turmeric powder, salt, and pepper. Cook for 3-4 minutes, stirring occasionally.
- ➢ Add spinach to the skillet and cook until wilted.
- ➢ Remove from heat and serve hot.

Health Benefits:

- ➢ Tofu is a great source of plant-based protein, providing all essential amino acids.

> Bell peppers and onions are rich in vitamins, minerals, and antioxidants, supporting overall health and immunity.

> Spinach adds extra fiber, vitamins, and minerals like iron and magnesium.

Preparation Time: 15 minutes

4. Overnight Oats

Ingredients:

> 1/2 cup rolled oats

> 1/2 cup almond milk or any plant-based milk

> 1 tablespoon chia seeds

> 1 tablespoon maple syrup or sweetener of choice

> Toppings: sliced fruits, nuts, seeds, nut butter

Instructions:

> In a mason jar or airtight container, combine rolled oats, almond milk, chia seeds, and maple syrup.

> Stir well to combine.

> Cover and refrigerate overnight, or for at least 4 hours.

- ➢ In the morning, give the oats a good stir and add more almond milk if desired to reach your desired consistency.
- ➢ Top with sliced fruits, nuts, seeds, and nut butter.
- ➢ Serve chilled.

Health Benefits:

- ➢ Oats are a good source of fiber, helping to regulate digestion and promote satiety.
- ➢ Chia seeds provide omega-3 fatty acids, protein, and additional fiber for heart health and satiety.
- ➢ Almond milk is low in calories and contains healthy fats and vitamin E.

Preparation Time: 5 minutes (plus overnight soaking)

5. Sweet Potato Breakfast Bowl

Ingredients:

- ➢ 1 small sweet potato, roasted
- ➢ 1/2 cup cooked quinoa
- ➢ 1/4 cup black beans, rinsed and drained
- ➢ 1/4 cup diced avocado
- ➢ Salsa or hot sauce (optional)

➢ Fresh cilantro for garnish

➢ Salt and pepper to taste

Instructions:

➢ Preheat the oven to 400°F (200°C). Pierce the sweet potato with a fork a few times, then place it on a baking sheet lined with parchment paper.

➢ Roast the sweet potato in the preheated oven for 45-60 minutes, or until tender.

➢ Once the sweet potato is cooked, remove it from the oven and let it cool slightly.

➢ Cut the sweet potato in half lengthwise and scoop out the flesh into a bowl.

➢ Top the sweet potato with cooked quinoa, black beans, diced avocado, salsa or hot sauce (if using), and fresh cilantro.

➢ Season with salt and pepper to taste.

➢ Serve warm.

Health Benefits:

➢ Sweet potatoes are rich in fiber, vitamins (such as vitamin A and C), and minerals (such as potassium), supporting digestion and immune function.

- ➢ Quinoa provides protein, fiber, and essential amino acids, promoting satiety and muscle repair.
- ➢ Black beans are a good source of plant-based protein, fiber, and antioxidants, supporting heart health and blood sugar control.

Preparation Time: 60 minutes

6. Vegan Banana Pancakes

Ingredients:

- ➢ 1 ripe banana, mashed
- ➢ 1/2 cup oat flour
- ➢ 1/4 cup almond milk or any plant-based milk
- ➢ 1 tablespoon maple syrup or sweetener of choice
- ➢ 1/2 teaspoon baking powder
- ➢ 1/2 teaspoon vanilla extract
- ➢ Pinch of salt
- ➢ Cooking oil for greasing the pan

Instructions:

- ➢ In a mixing bowl, combine mashed banana, oat flour, almond milk, maple syrup, baking powder, vanilla extract, and a pinch of salt. Stir until well combined and smooth.

- ➤ Heat a non-stick skillet or griddle over medium heat and lightly grease with cooking oil.
- ➤ Pour a small amount of pancake batter onto the skillet to form pancakes of desired size.
- ➤ Cook for 2-3 minutes, or until bubbles form on the surface of the pancakes.
- ➤ Flip the pancakes and cook for an additional 1-2 minutes, or until golden brown and cooked through.
- ➤ Repeat with the remaining batter.
- ➤ Serve warm with toppings of choice, such as sliced fruits, nuts, seeds, and maple syrup.

Health Benefits:

- ➤ Bananas are rich in potassium, fiber, and natural sugars, providing energy and supporting muscle function.
- ➤ Oat flour is gluten-free and high in fiber, promoting satiety and digestive health.
- ➤ Almond milk is low in calories and contains healthy fats and vitamin E.

Preparation Time: 15 minutes

7. Chia Pudding

Ingredients:

- ➤ 1/4 cup chia seeds
- ➤ 1 cup almond milk or any plant-based milk
- ➤ 1 tablespoon maple syrup or sweetener of choice
- ➤ 1/2 teaspoon vanilla extract
- ➤ Toppings: sliced fruits, nuts, seeds, coconut flakes

Instructions:

- ➤ In a mason jar or airtight container, combine chia seeds, almond milk, maple syrup, and vanilla extract.
- ➤ Stir well to combine.
- ➤ Cover and refrigerate for at least 2 hours, or overnight, until the mixture thickens and forms a pudding-like consistency.
- ➤ Once the chia pudding is ready, give it a good stir.
- ➤ Serve chilled with toppings of choice, such as sliced fruits, nuts, seeds, and coconut flakes.

Health Benefits:

> Chia seeds are rich in omega-3 fatty acids, protein, and fiber, promoting heart health, satiety, and digestive health.
> Almond milk is low in calories and contains healthy fats and vitamin E.

Preparation Time: 5 minutes (plus chilling time)

8. Veggie Breakfast Burrito

Ingredients:

> 1 whole grain tortilla or wrap
> 1/2 cup tofu scramble (see recipe #3)
> 1/4 cup black beans, rinsed and drained
> 1/4 cup diced avocado
> Salsa or hot sauce (optional)
> Fresh cilantro for garnish
> Salt and pepper to taste

Instructions:

> Heat the tortilla or wrap in a skillet or microwave until warm and pliable.

➢ Spread tofu scramble onto the tortilla, leaving space around the edges.

➢ Top with black beans, diced avocado, salsa or hot sauce (if using), and fresh cilantro.

➢ Season with salt and pepper to taste.

➢ Fold in the sides of the tortilla and roll it up tightly to form a burrito.

➢ Serve immediately.

Health Benefits:

➢ Tofu provides plant-based protein and essential amino acids, supporting muscle repair and satiety.

➢ Black beans are a good source of protein, fiber, and antioxidants, promoting heart health and blood sugar control.

➢ Avocado adds healthy fats, fiber, and vitamins, supporting heart health and satiety.

Preparation Time: 15 minutes (if tofu scramble is pre-made)

9. Green Smoothie

Ingredients:

➢ 1 cup spinach or kale leaves

- ➢ 1/2 frozen banana
- ➢ 1/2 cup frozen mixed berries
- ➢ 1/4 avocado
- ➢ 1 tablespoon chia seeds
- ➢ 1 cup almond milk or any plant-based milk
- ➢ Optional: 1 tablespoon nut butter or protein powder

Instructions:

- ➢ In a blender, combine spinach or kale leaves, frozen banana, frozen mixed berries, avocado, chia seeds, almond milk, and optional nut butter or protein powder.
- ➢ Blend until smooth and creamy, adding more almond milk if needed to reach your desired consistency.
- ➢ Pour the smoothie into a glass.
- ➢ Serve immediately.

Health Benefits:

- ➢ Spinach or kale adds fiber, vitamins, and minerals like iron and calcium.
- ➢ Berries are packed with antioxidants, vitamins, and fiber, supporting digestion and immune function.

> Chia seeds provide omega-3 fatty acids, protein, and additional fiber for heart health and satiety.

Preparation Time: 5 minutes

10. Peanut Butter Banana Toast

Ingredients:

> 2 slices of whole grain bread
>
> 2 tablespoons peanut butter
>
> 1 ripe banana, sliced
>
> Optional: drizzle of honey or maple syrup

Instructions:

> Toast the bread slices until golden brown.
>
> Spread peanut butter evenly onto the toasted bread slices.
>
> Top with sliced banana.
>
> Optional: Drizzle honey or maple syrup over the banana slices for extra sweetness.
>
> Serve immediately.

Health Benefits:

> ➢ Peanut butter provides plant-based protein, healthy fats, and essential nutrients like vitamin E and magnesium.
> ➢ Bananas are rich in potassium, fiber, and natural sugars, providing energy and supporting muscle function.

Preparation Time: 5 minutes

Plant Based Weight Loss Lunch Recipes

1. Quinoa Salad with Chickpeas and Avocado

Ingredients:

> ➢ 1 cup cooked quinoa
> ➢ 1/2 cup cooked chickpeas (canned is fine)
> ➢ 1/2 ripe avocado, diced
> ➢ 1/4 cup diced cucumber
> ➢ 1/4 cup diced bell pepper
> ➢ Handful of cherry tomatoes, halved
> ➢ Fresh parsley or cilantro, chopped
> ➢ Juice of 1 lemon
> ➢ Salt and pepper to taste

Instructions:

> In a large mixing bowl, combine cooked quinoa, chickpeas, avocado, cucumber, bell pepper, and cherry tomatoes.
> Drizzle lemon juice over the salad and toss gently to combine.
> Season with salt and pepper to taste.
> Garnish with fresh parsley or cilantro.
> Serve chilled or at room temperature.

Health Benefits:

> Quinoa provides protein, fiber, and essential amino acids, supporting muscle repair and satiety.
> Chickpeas are rich in plant-based protein, fiber, and vitamins, promoting heart health and blood sugar control.
> Avocado adds healthy fats, fiber, and vitamins, supporting heart health and satiety.

Preparation Time: 15 minutes

2. Lentil Soup

Ingredients:

- 1 cup dried lentils, rinsed and drained
- 1 onion, diced
- 2 carrots, diced
- 2 celery stalks, diced
- 2 garlic cloves, minced
- 4 cups vegetable broth
- 1 can diced tomatoes
- 1 teaspoon ground cumin
- 1 teaspoon ground coriander
- Salt and pepper to taste
- Fresh parsley for garnish (optional)

Instructions:

- In a large pot, sauté onion, carrots, celery, and garlic in a little bit of olive oil until softened.
- Add dried lentils, vegetable broth, diced tomatoes, ground cumin, and ground coriander to the pot.
- Bring the soup to a boil, then reduce heat and simmer for 20-25 minutes, or until lentils are tender.
- Season with salt and pepper to taste.

➢ Garnish with fresh parsley before serving, if desired.

➢ Serve hot.

Health Benefits:

➢ Lentils are a good source of plant-based protein, fiber, and minerals like iron and folate, supporting muscle repair and heart health.

➢ Vegetables like carrots, celery, and tomatoes add vitamins, minerals, and antioxidants, supporting overall health and immunity.

Preparation Time: 30 minutes

3. Chickpea Salad Sandwich

Ingredients:

➢ 1 can chickpeas, rinsed and drained

➢ 2 tablespoons vegan mayonnaise

➢ 1 tablespoon Dijon mustard

➢ 1 stalk celery, diced

➢ 1/4 cup diced red onion

➢ 1/4 cup chopped pickles

➢ Salt and pepper to taste

➢ Whole grain bread or lettuce leaves for serving

Instructions:

- ➤ In a mixing bowl, mash chickpeas with a fork or potato masher until chunky.
- ➤ Add vegan mayonnaise, Dijon mustard, diced celery, red onion, chopped pickles, salt, and pepper to the mashed chickpeas. Mix until well combined.
- ➤ Adjust seasoning to taste.
- ➤ Serve the chickpea salad on whole grain bread slices or lettuce leaves to make sandwiches.
- ➤ Serve immediately.

Health Benefits:

- ➤ Chickpeas provide plant-based protein, fiber, and vitamins, supporting muscle repair and satiety.
- ➤ Celery, red onion, and pickles add crunch, flavor, and additional fiber and antioxidants.

Preparation Time: 10 minutes

4. Mediterranean Quinoa Bowl

Ingredients:

- ➤ 1 cup cooked quinoa
- ➤ 1/2 cup chickpeas, rinsed and drained

- ➢ 1/4 cup sliced cucumber
- ➢ 1/4 cup cherry tomatoes, halved
- ➢ 1/4 cup sliced Kalamata olives
- ➢ 2 tablespoons crumbled feta cheese (optional)
- ➢ Fresh parsley or basil, chopped
- ➢ Juice of 1 lemon
- ➢ Extra virgin olive oil
- ➢ Salt and pepper to taste

Instructions:

- ➢ In a mixing bowl, combine cooked quinoa, chickpeas, cucumber, cherry tomatoes, Kalamata olives, and crumbled feta cheese (if using).
- ➢ Drizzle lemon juice and olive oil over the quinoa bowl.
- ➢ Season with salt and pepper to taste.
- ➢ Garnish with fresh parsley or basil.
- ➢ Serve chilled or at room temperature.

Health Benefits:

- ➢ Quinoa provides protein, fiber, and essential amino acids, supporting muscle repair and satiety.

> Chickpeas are rich in plant-based protein, fiber, and vitamins, promoting heart health and blood sugar control.

> Mediterranean ingredients like olives and olive oil add healthy fats, antioxidants, and flavor.

Preparation Time: 15 minutes

5. Vegan Buddha Bowl

Ingredients:

> 1 cup cooked brown rice or quinoa

> 1/2 cup cooked black beans (canned is fine)

> 1/2 cup roasted sweet potatoes, cubed

> 1/2 cup steamed broccoli florets

> 1/4 cup shredded carrots

> 1/4 avocado, sliced

> 1 tablespoon tahini

> 1 tablespoon soy sauce or tamari

> 1 teaspoon maple syrup

> 1 teaspoon sriracha (optional)

> Sesame seeds for garnish

Instructions:

- Arrange cooked brown rice or quinoa, black beans, roasted sweet potatoes, steamed broccoli florets, shredded carrots, and sliced avocado in a bowl.
- In a small bowl, whisk together tahini, soy sauce or tamari, maple syrup, and sriracha (if using) to make the dressing.
- Drizzle the dressing over the Buddha bowl.
- Garnish with sesame seeds.
- Serve immediately.

Health Benefits:

- Brown rice or quinoa provides complex carbohydrates, protein, and essential nutrients like B vitamins and minerals.
- Black beans are a good source of plant-based protein, fiber, and antioxidants, supporting heart health and blood sugar control.
- Vegetables like sweet potatoes, broccoli, carrots, and avocado add vitamins, minerals, fiber, and antioxidants.

Preparation Time: 30 minutes

6. Stuffed Bell Peppers

Ingredients:

- ➢ 2 large bell peppers, halved and seeds removed
- ➢ 1 cup cooked quinoa or brown rice
- ➢ 1/2 cup black beans, rinsed and drained
- ➢ 1/2 cup corn kernels (fresh or frozen)
- ➢ 1/4 cup diced tomatoes
- ➢ 1/4 cup diced red onion
- ➢ 1/4 cup chopped cilantro
- ➢ 1 teaspoon ground cumin
- ➢ 1 teaspoon chili powder
- ➢ Salt and pepper to taste
- ➢ Optional toppings: avocado slices, salsa, vegan cheese

Instructions:

- ➢ Preheat the oven to 375°F (190°C).
- ➢ In a mixing bowl, combine cooked quinoa or brown rice, black beans, corn kernels, diced tomatoes, red onion, chopped cilantro, ground cumin, chili powder, salt, and pepper.

- ➢ Stuff the halved bell peppers with the quinoa mixture.
- ➢ Place the stuffed bell peppers in a baking dish.
- ➢ Cover the dish with aluminum foil and bake in the preheated oven for 25-30 minutes, or until the bell peppers are tender.
- ➢ Remove from the oven and let cool slightly before serving.
- ➢ Top with optional toppings like avocado slices, salsa, or vegan cheese, if desired.
- ➢ Serve hot.

Health Benefits:

- ➢ Bell peppers are rich in vitamins (such as vitamin C and vitamin A), minerals, and antioxidants, supporting overall health and immunity.
- ➢ Quinoa or brown rice provides complex carbohydrates, protein, and essential nutrients like B vitamins and minerals.
- ➢ Black beans add plant-based protein, fiber, and antioxidants, promoting heart health and blood sugar control.

Preparation Time: 45 minutes

7. Chickpea and Vegetable Stir-Fry

Ingredients:

- ➢ 1 can chickpeas, rinsed and drained
- ➢ 2 cups mixed vegetables (such as bell peppers, broccoli, carrots, snap peas)
- ➢ 2 garlic cloves, minced
- ➢ 1-inch piece of ginger, minced
- ➢ 2 tablespoons soy sauce or tamari
- ➢ 1 tablespoon rice vinegar
- ➢ 1 tablespoon maple syrup
- ➢ 1 teaspoon cornstarch (optional)
- ➢ 1 tablespoon sesame oil
- ➢ Cooked brown rice or quinoa for serving

Instructions:

- ➢ In a small bowl, whisk together soy sauce or tamari, rice vinegar, maple syrup, and cornstarch (if using) to make the sauce. Set aside.
- ➢ Heat sesame oil in a large skillet or wok over medium-high heat.

- ➤ Add minced garlic and ginger to the skillet, and sauté for 1-2 minutes until fragrant.
- ➤ Add mixed vegetables to the skillet and stir-fry for 5-7 minutes until tender-crisp.
- ➤ Add chickpeas and the prepared sauce to the skillet, and cook for another 2-3 minutes until heated through and the sauce has thickened slightly.
- ➤ Remove from heat.
- ➤ Serve the chickpea and vegetable stir-fry over cooked brown rice or quinoa.
- ➤ Serve hot.

Health Benefits:

- ➤ Chickpeas provide plant-based protein, fiber, and vitamins, promoting muscle repair and satiety.
- ➤ Mixed vegetables add vitamins, minerals, fiber, and antioxidants, supporting overall health and immunity.

Preparation Time: 20 minutes

8. Vegan Lentil Salad

Ingredients:

- ➤ 1 cup cooked lentils
- ➤ 1/2 cucumber, diced
- ➤ 1/2 bell pepper, diced
- ➤ 1/4 red onion, thinly sliced
- ➤ 1/4 cup cherry tomatoes, halved
- ➤ Handful of fresh parsley, chopped
- ➤ Juice of 1 lemon
- ➤ 2 tablespoons extra virgin olive oil
- ➤ Salt and pepper to taste

Instructions:

- ➤ In a mixing bowl, combine cooked lentils, diced cucumber, bell pepper, red onion, cherry tomatoes, and chopped parsley.
- ➤ Drizzle lemon juice and extra virgin olive oil over the lentil salad.
- ➤ Season with salt and pepper to taste.
- ➤ Toss gently to combine.
- ➤ Serve chilled or at room temperature.

Health Benefits:

> Lentils provide plant-based protein, fiber, and essential nutrients like iron and folate, supporting muscle repair and blood health.

> Vegetables like cucumber, bell pepper, red onion, and cherry tomatoes add vitamins, minerals, fiber, and antioxidants.

Preparation Time: 15 minutes

9. Vegan Falafel Wrap

Ingredients:

> 4-6 store-bought or homemade falafel patties

> 2 whole grain wraps or tortillas

> 1/4 cup hummus

> 1/2 cup shredded lettuce

> 1/4 cup diced tomatoes

> 1/4 cup sliced cucumber

> 2 tablespoons tahini sauce or dressing

> Fresh parsley for garnish (optional)

Instructions:

- ➤ Heat the falafel patties according to package instructions, if using store-bought.
- ➤ Warm the wraps or tortillas in a skillet or microwave until pliable.
- ➤ Spread hummus onto each wrap or tortilla.
- ➤ Place 2-3 falafel patties on each wrap or tortilla.
- ➤ Top with shredded lettuce, diced tomatoes, sliced cucumber, and drizzle with tahini sauce or dressing.
- ➤ Garnish with fresh parsley, if desired.
- ➤ Roll up the wraps tightly.
- ➤ Serve immediately.

Health Benefits:

- ➤ Falafel provides plant-based protein, fiber, and essential nutrients like iron and magnesium, supporting muscle repair and energy production.
- ➤ Hummus adds protein, healthy fats, and fiber, promoting satiety and heart health.
- ➤ Vegetables like lettuce, tomatoes, and cucumber add vitamins, minerals, fiber, and antioxidants.

Preparation Time: 15 minutes

10. Veggie Sushi Rolls

Ingredients:

- ➢ 2 nori seaweed sheets
- ➢ 1 cup cooked sushi rice
- ➢ 1/2 avocado, sliced
- ➢ 1/4 cucumber, julienned
- ➢ 1/4 bell pepper, julienned
- ➢ 1/4 carrot, julienned
- ➢ 2-3 tablespoons pickled ginger
- ➢ 2-3 tablespoons low-sodium soy sauce or tamari
- ➢ Wasabi and/or vegan mayo for dipping (optional)

Instructions:

- ➢ Place a nori seaweed sheet on a bamboo sushi mat or clean kitchen towel.
- ➢ Spread a thin layer of cooked sushi rice evenly over the nori seaweed sheet, leaving a small border along the edges.
- ➢ Arrange avocado slices, julienned cucumber, bell pepper, and carrot in the center of the rice.
- ➢ Add a few pieces of pickled ginger on top of the vegetables.

- Using the bamboo sushi mat or towel, roll the nori seaweed sheet tightly into a sushi roll.
- Repeat with the remaining ingredients to make a second sushi roll.
- Use a sharp knife to slice each sushi roll into 6-8 pieces.
- Serve the veggie sushi rolls with low-sodium soy sauce or tamari for dipping, and wasabi and/or vegan mayo if desired.
- Serve immediately.

Health Benefits:

- Nori seaweed sheets are rich in iodine, vitamins, minerals, and antioxidants, supporting thyroid health and overall well-being.
- Sushi rice provides carbohydrates for energy and essential nutrients like manganese and selenium.
- Vegetables like avocado, cucumber, bell pepper, and carrot add vitamins, minerals, fiber, and antioxidants.

Preparation Time: 30 minutes

1. Quinoa Stuffed Bell Peppers

Ingredients:

- 4 large bell peppers, any color
- 1 cup cooked quinoa
- 1 can (15 oz) black beans, drained and rinsed
- 1 cup corn kernels (fresh, frozen, or canned)
- 1 cup diced tomatoes
- 1/2 cup diced onion
- 2 cloves garlic, minced
- 1 teaspoon cumin
- 1 teaspoon chili powder
- Salt and pepper to taste
- Optional toppings: avocado slices, chopped cilantro, salsa

Instructions:

- Preheat the oven to 375°F (190°C).
- Cut the tops off the bell peppers and remove the seeds and membranes. Place the peppers upright in a baking dish.

- In a large mixing bowl, combine cooked quinoa, black beans, corn, diced tomatoes, onion, garlic, cumin, chili powder, salt, and pepper. Mix until well combined.
- Spoon the quinoa mixture into each bell pepper until they are filled to the top.
- Cover the baking dish with foil and bake in the preheated oven for 30-35 minutes, or until the peppers are tender.
- Remove from the oven and let cool slightly before serving.
- Garnish with optional toppings such as avocado slices, chopped cilantro, and salsa.
- Serve hot.

Health Benefits:

- Bell peppers are rich in vitamins A and C, antioxidants, and fiber, supporting immune function and digestion.
- Quinoa provides protein, fiber, and essential amino acids, promoting satiety and muscle repair.

> Black beans are a good source of plant-based protein, fiber, and antioxidants, supporting heart health and blood sugar control.

Preparation Time: 45 minutes

2. Lentil and Vegetable Soup

Ingredients:

> 1 cup dry green or brown lentils, rinsed

> 6 cups vegetable broth or water

> 1 onion, diced

> 2 carrots, diced

> 2 celery stalks, diced

> 2 cloves garlic, minced

> 1 can (15 oz) diced tomatoes

> 2 cups chopped spinach or kale

> 1 teaspoon dried thyme

> 1 teaspoon dried oregano

> Salt and pepper to taste

> Optional toppings: fresh parsley, lemon wedges

Instructions:

> - In a large pot, combine lentils, vegetable broth or water, onion, carrots, celery, garlic, diced tomatoes, thyme, and oregano. Bring to a boil.
> - Reduce heat to low and simmer for 25-30 minutes, or until lentils and vegetables are tender.
> - Stir in chopped spinach or kale and cook for an additional 5 minutes, until wilted.
> - Season with salt and pepper to taste.
> - Remove from heat and let cool slightly before serving.
> - Garnish with fresh parsley and lemon wedges, if desired.
> - Serve hot.

Health Benefits:

> - Lentils are high in protein, fiber, and iron, promoting satiety, digestive health, and energy levels.
> - Vegetables like carrots, celery, and spinach are rich in vitamins, minerals, and antioxidants, supporting overall health and immunity.

Preparation Time: 40 minutes

Ingredients:

- ➢ 1 tablespoon coconut oil or olive oil
- ➢ 1 onion, diced
- ➢ 3 cloves garlic, minced
- ➢ 1 tablespoon grated ginger
- ➢ 2 teaspoons curry powder
- ➢ 1 teaspoon ground cumin
- ➢ 1/2 teaspoon turmeric powder
- ➢ 1 can (15 oz) chickpeas, drained and rinsed
- ➢ 1 can (14 oz) coconut milk
- ➢ 1 cup diced tomatoes
- ➢ 2 cups chopped spinach or kale
- ➢ Salt and pepper to taste
- ➢ Cooked brown rice or quinoa for serving
- ➢ Optional toppings: fresh cilantro, lime wedges

Instructions:

- ➢ Heat coconut oil or olive oil in a large skillet over medium heat.
- ➢ Add diced onion, minced garlic, and grated ginger to the skillet. Sauté for 2-3 minutes, until fragrant.

- ➢ Stir in curry powder, ground cumin, and turmeric powder. Cook for an additional 1-2 minutes.
- ➢ Add chickpeas, coconut milk, and diced tomatoes to the skillet. Bring to a simmer and cook for 10-15 minutes, stirring occasionally.
- ➢ Stir in chopped spinach or kale and cook until wilted.
- ➢ Season with salt and pepper to taste.
- ➢ Serve the chickpea curry over cooked brown rice or quinoa.
- ➢ Garnish with fresh cilantro and lime wedges, if desired.
- ➢ Serve hot.

Health Benefits:

- ➢ Chickpeas are a good source of plant-based protein, fiber, and iron, supporting muscle repair, satiety, and energy levels.
- ➢ Coconut milk provides healthy fats and adds richness and creaminess to the curry.
- ➢ Spinach or kale adds extra fiber, vitamins, and minerals like iron and calcium.

Preparation Time: 30 minutes

4. Vegetable Stir-Fry

Ingredients:

- ➢ 2 cups mixed vegetables (such as bell peppers, broccoli, carrots, snap peas, mushrooms)
- ➢ 1 tablespoon sesame oil or olive oil
- ➢ 2 cloves garlic, minced
- ➢ 1 tablespoon grated ginger
- ➢ 1/4 cup low-sodium soy sauce or tamari
- ➢ 2 tablespoons rice vinegar
- ➢ 1 tablespoon maple syrup or sweetener of choice
- ➢ 2 cups cooked brown rice or quinoa
- ➢ Optional toppings: sliced green onions, sesame seeds

Instructions:

- ➢ Heat sesame oil or olive oil in a large skillet or wok over medium-high heat.
- ➢ Add mixed vegetables to the skillet and stir-fry for 5-7 minutes, until tender-crisp.
- ➢ Stir in minced garlic and grated ginger, and cook for an additional 1-2 minutes, until fragrant.
- ➢ In a small bowl, whisk together soy sauce or tamari, rice vinegar, and maple syrup.

- Pour the sauce over the vegetables in the skillet and toss to coat evenly.
- Cook for an additional 2-3 minutes, until the sauce thickens slightly.
- Serve the vegetable stir-fry over cooked brown rice or quinoa.
- Garnish with sliced green onions and sesame seeds, if desired.
- Serve hot.

Health Benefits:

- Mixed vegetables provide vitamins, minerals, and antioxidants, supporting overall health and immunity.
- Brown rice or quinoa adds fiber, protein, and essential nutrients, promoting satiety and muscle repair.
- Sesame oil adds flavor and healthy fats, while ginger and garlic provide anti-inflammatory and immune-boosting properties.

Preparation Time: 20 minutes

5. Spaghetti Squash with Marinara Sauce

Ingredients:

- ➢ 1 medium spaghetti squash
- ➢ 2 cups marinara sauce (homemade or store-bought)
- ➢ Optional toppings: nutritional yeast, fresh basil leaves

Instructions:

- ➢ Preheat the oven to 400°F (200°C).
- ➢ Cut the spaghetti squash in half lengthwise and scoop out the seeds.
- ➢ Place the squash halves cut side down on a baking sheet lined with parchment paper.
- ➢ Bake in the preheated oven for 30-40 minutes, or until the squash is tender and easily pierced with a fork.
- ➢ Remove from the oven and let cool slightly.
- ➢ Use a fork to scrape the flesh of the squash into spaghetti-like strands.
- ➢ Heat marinara sauce in a saucepan over medium heat until warmed through.
- ➢ Serve the spaghetti squash with marinara sauce.

- ➢ Garnish with optional toppings such as nutritional yeast and fresh basil leaves.
- ➢ Serve hot.

Health Benefits:

- ➢ Spaghetti squash is low in calories and carbohydrates, making it a lighter alternative to traditional pasta.
- ➢ Marinara sauce provides vitamins, minerals, and antioxidants from tomatoes, garlic, and herbs.
- ➢ Nutritional yeast adds a cheesy flavor and is a good source of B vitamins and protein.

Preparation Time: 45 minutes

6. Black Bean Tacos

Ingredients:

- ➢ 1 can (15 oz) black beans, drained and rinsed
- ➢ 1/2 cup diced tomatoes
- ➢ 1/4 cup diced onion
- ➢ 1 teaspoon chili powder
- ➢ 1/2 teaspoon cumin
- ➢ Salt and pepper to taste

- ➢ 8 small corn or whole grain tortillas
- ➢ Toppings: shredded lettuce, diced avocado, salsa, lime wedges

Instructions:

- ➢ In a medium saucepan, combine black beans, diced tomatoes, diced onion, chili powder, cumin, salt, and pepper.
- ➢ Cook over medium heat for 5-7 minutes, stirring occasionally, until heated through and flavors are combined.
- ➢ Warm tortillas in a skillet or microwave until soft and pliable.
- ➢ Spoon black bean mixture onto each tortilla.
- ➢ Top with shredded lettuce, diced avocado, salsa, and a squeeze of lime juice.
- ➢ Fold or roll up the tacos and serve immediately.

Health Benefits:

- ➢ Black beans are a good source of plant-based protein, fiber, and antioxidants, supporting heart health and blood sugar control.

- ➢ Tomatoes and onions provide vitamins, minerals, and antioxidants, supporting overall health and immunity.
- ➢ Avocado adds healthy fats, fiber, and vitamins, promoting satiety and heart health.

Preparation Time: 15 minutes

7. Vegan Lentil Shepherd's Pie

Ingredients:

- ➢ 2 cups cooked green or brown lentils
- ➢ 1 onion, diced
- ➢ 2 carrots, diced
- ➢ 2 celery stalks, diced
- ➢ 2 cloves garlic, minced
- ➢ 1 cup frozen peas
- ➢ 1 cup vegetable broth
- ➢ 2 tablespoons tomato paste
- ➢ 1 tablespoon soy sauce or tamari
- ➢ 1 teaspoon dried thyme
- ➢ 1 teaspoon dried rosemary
- ➢ Salt and pepper to taste
- ➢ 4 cups mashed potatoes (homemade or store-bought)

- Optional: vegan cheese for topping

Instructions:

- Preheat the oven to 375°F (190°C).
- In a large skillet, heat oil over medium heat. Add diced onion, carrots, and celery, and sauté until softened, about 5-7 minutes.
- Add minced garlic and cook for an additional 1-2 minutes, until fragrant.
- Stir in cooked lentils, frozen peas, vegetable broth, tomato paste, soy sauce, dried thyme, dried rosemary, salt, and pepper. Cook for 5-7 minutes, until heated through and flavors are combined.
- Transfer the lentil mixture to a baking dish and spread it out evenly.
- Top with mashed potatoes, spreading them out evenly over the lentil mixture.
- Optional: Sprinkle vegan cheese on top of the mashed potatoes.
- Bake in the preheated oven for 25-30 minutes, or until the mashed potatoes are golden brown and the filling is bubbly.

- ➢ Remove from the oven and let cool slightly before serving.
- ➢ Serve hot.

Health Benefits:

- ➢ Lentils are a good source of plant-based protein, fiber, and iron, supporting muscle repair, satiety, and energy levels.
- ➢ Vegetables like onions, carrots, celery, and peas provide vitamins, minerals, and antioxidants, supporting overall health and immunity.
- ➢ Mashed potatoes add comfort and satisfaction to the dish while providing carbohydrates for energy.

Preparation Time: 60 minutes

8. Vegetable and Tofu Stir-Fry

Ingredients:

- ➢ 1 block firm tofu, drained and pressed
- ➢ 2 tablespoons soy sauce or tamari
- ➢ 1 tablespoon cornstarch
- ➢ 1 tablespoon sesame oil or olive oil

- 2 cups mixed vegetables (such as bell peppers, broccoli, carrots, snap peas, mushrooms)
- 2 cloves garlic, minced
- 1 tablespoon grated ginger
- Cooked brown rice or quinoa for serving
- Optional toppings: sliced green onions, sesame seeds

Instructions:

- Cut pressed tofu into cubes and place them in a mixing bowl.
- In a small bowl, whisk together soy sauce or tamari and cornstarch until smooth. Pour the mixture over the tofu cubes and toss to coat evenly.
- Heat sesame oil or olive oil in a large skillet or wok over medium-high heat.
- Add tofu cubes to the skillet and cook for 5-7 minutes, stirring occasionally, until golden brown and crispy.
- Remove tofu from the skillet and set aside.
- In the same skillet, add mixed vegetables and stir-fry for 5-7 minutes, until tender-crisp.
- Add minced garlic and grated ginger to the skillet and cook for an additional 1-2 minutes, until fragrant.

- Return cooked tofu to the skillet and toss to combine with the vegetables.
- Serve the vegetable and tofu stir-fry over cooked brown rice or quinoa.
- Garnish with sliced green onions and sesame seeds, if desired.
- Serve hot.

Health Benefits:

- Tofu provides plant-based protein, calcium, and essential amino acids, supporting muscle repair, bone health, and satiety.
- Mixed vegetables provide vitamins, minerals, and antioxidants, supporting overall health and immunity.
- Brown rice or quinoa adds fiber, protein, and essential nutrients, promoting satiety and muscle repair.

Preparation Time: 30 minutes

9. Mediterranean Chickpea Salad

Ingredients:

- ➤ 1 can (15 oz) chickpeas, drained and rinsed
- ➤ 1 cup diced cucumber
- ➤ 1 cup cherry tomatoes, halved
- ➤ 1/4 cup diced red onion
- ➤ 1/4 cup chopped fresh parsley
- ➤ 2 tablespoons lemon juice
- ➤ 2 tablespoons extra-virgin olive oil
- ➤ 1 clove garlic, minced
- ➤ 1 teaspoon dried oregano
- ➤ Salt and pepper to taste
- ➤ Optional toppings: crumbled feta cheese, olives, chopped fresh mint

Instructions:

- ➤ In a large mixing bowl, combine chickpeas, diced cucumber, cherry tomatoes, diced red onion, and chopped parsley.
- ➤ In a small bowl, whisk together lemon juice, olive oil, minced garlic, dried oregano, salt, and pepper.

➢ Pour the dressing over the chickpea mixture and toss to coat evenly.

➢ Let the salad marinates in the refrigerator for at least 30 minutes to allow the flavors to meld.

➢ Just before serving, garnish the salad with optional toppings such as crumbled feta cheese, olives, and chopped fresh mint.

➢ Serve chilled or at room temperature.

Health Benefits:

➢ Chickpeas are a good source of plant-based protein, fiber, and antioxidants, supporting heart health, digestion, and blood sugar control.

➢ Vegetables like cucumber, tomatoes, and onions provide vitamins, minerals, and antioxidants, supporting overall health and immunity.

➢ Olive oil adds healthy fats and anti-inflammatory properties, while lemon juice provides vitamin C and acidity to brighten the flavors of the salad.

Preparation Time: 15 minutes

Ingredients:

- 1 tablespoon coconut oil or olive oil
- 1 onion, diced
- 2 cloves garlic, minced
- 1 tablespoon grated ginger
- 2 tablespoons curry powder
- 1 teaspoon ground turmeric
- 1 can (14 oz) coconut milk
- 2 cups mixed vegetables (such as bell peppers, broccoli, carrots, snap peas, mushrooms)
- Salt and pepper to taste
- Cooked brown rice or quinoa for serving
- Optional toppings: chopped fresh cilantro, lime wedges

Instructions:

- Heat coconut oil or olive oil in a large skillet or pot over medium heat.
- Add diced onion to the skillet and sauté for 5-7 minutes, until softened.

- Stir in minced garlic, grated ginger, curry powder, and ground turmeric. Cook for an additional 1-2 minutes, until fragrant.
- Add coconut milk to the skillet and stir to combine with the onion and spice mixture.
- Bring the mixture to a simmer and cook for 5 minutes.
- Add mixed vegetables to the skillet and simmer for 10-15 minutes, until vegetables are tender.
- Season with salt and pepper to taste.
- Serve the vegetable curry over cooked brown rice or quinoa.
- Garnish with chopped fresh cilantro and lime wedges, if desired.
- Serve hot.

Health Benefits:

- Coconut milk adds creaminess and richness to the curry while providing healthy fats and anti-inflammatory properties.
- Mixed vegetables provide vitamins, minerals, and antioxidants, supporting overall health and immunity.

> Brown rice or quinoa adds fiber, protein, and
> essential nutrients, promoting satiety and muscle
> repair.

Preparation Time: 30 minutes

Plant Based Weight Loss Snacks Recipes

1. Hummus and Veggie Sticks

Ingredients:

> 1/4 cup hummus (store-bought or homemade)
> Assorted vegetable sticks (carrots, cucumber, bell
> peppers, celery)

Instructions:

> Place hummus in a small bowl.
> Wash and chop vegetables into sticks.
> Dip veggie sticks into hummus and enjoy!

Health Benefits:

> Hummus provides plant-based protein and healthy
> fats, while vegetables offer fiber, vitamins, and
> minerals, supporting overall health and satiety.

Preparation Time: 5 minutes

2. Trail Mix

Ingredients:

> ➤ 1/4 cup almonds
>
> ➤ 1/4 cup walnuts
>
> ➤ 1/4 cup pumpkin seeds
>
> ➤ 1/4 cup dried cranberries or raisins

Instructions:

> ➤ Mix all ingredients in a bowl.
>
> ➤ Portion into individual snack-sized bags for easy grab-and-go options.

Health Benefits:

> ➤ Nuts and seeds provide healthy fats, protein, and fiber, while dried fruits offer natural sweetness and additional nutrients like vitamins and minerals.

Preparation Time: 5 minutes

3. Rice Cake with Almond Butter and Banana Slices

Ingredients:

> ➤ 1 rice cake

- ➢ 1 tablespoon almond butter
- ➢ 1/2 banana, sliced

Instructions:

- ➢ Spread almond butter onto the rice cake.
- ➢ Top with banana slices.
- ➢ Serve immediately.

Health Benefits:

- ➢ Rice cakes are low in calories and provide a crunchy base, while almond butter offers protein, healthy fats, and vitamins. Bananas add natural sweetness and potassium.

Preparation Time: 3 minutes

4. Guacamole and Whole Grain Crackers

Ingredients:

- ➢ 1 ripe avocado
- ➢ 1/2 lime, juiced
- ➢ 1/4 teaspoon salt
- ➢ 1/4 teaspoon pepper
- ➢ Whole grain crackers

Instructions:

> ➤ Mash the avocado in a bowl.
> ➤ Add lime juice, salt, and pepper, and mix until well combined.
> ➤ Serve with whole grain crackers for dipping.

Health Benefits:

> ➤ Avocado provides healthy fats and fiber, while whole grain crackers offer complex carbohydrates and additional fiber.

Preparation Time: 5 minutes

5. Energy Balls

Ingredients:

> ➤ 1 cup rolled oats
> ➤ 1/2 cup almond butter
> ➤ 1/4 cup maple syrup or honey
> ➤ 1/4 cup shredded coconut
> ➤ 1/4 cup dark chocolate chips

Instructions:

> In a mixing bowl, combine rolled oats, almond butter, maple syrup or honey, shredded coconut, and dark chocolate chips.
> Mix until well combined.
> Roll the mixture into small balls.
> Place energy balls on a baking sheet lined with parchment paper and refrigerate until firm.
> Store in an airtight container in the refrigerator.

Health Benefits:

> Energy balls are a convenient and portable snack option, providing a balance of carbohydrates, protein, and healthy fats.
> Oats offer fiber and sustained energy, while almond butter and dark chocolate chips add protein and antioxidants.

Preparation Time: 15 minutes

6. Veggie Sushi Rolls

Ingredients:

> Nori sheets

- ➢ Cooked quinoa or brown rice
- ➢ Assorted vegetables (cucumber, avocado, bell peppers, carrots)
- ➢ Soy sauce or tamari (for dipping)

Instructions:

- ➢ Place a nori sheet on a clean surface.
- ➢ Spread a thin layer of cooked quinoa or brown rice over the nori sheet.
- ➢ Arrange sliced vegetables on top of the rice.
- ➢ Roll the nori sheet tightly, using a sushi mat or your hands.
- ➢ Slice the sushi roll into bite-sized pieces.
- ➢ Serve with soy sauce or tamari for dipping.

Health Benefits:

- ➢ Veggie sushi rolls are low in calories and provide a combination of complex carbohydrates, fiber, and vitamins from the vegetables, supporting satiety and overall health.

Preparation Time: 15 minutes

7. Apple Slices with Nut Butter

Ingredients:

> ➤ 1 apple, sliced

> ➤ 2 tablespoons almond butter or peanut butter

Instructions:

> ➤ Slice the apple into thin slices.

> ➤ Spread nut butter onto each apple slice.

> ➤ Serve immediately.

Health Benefits:

> ➤ Apples are rich in fiber, vitamins, and antioxidants, while nut butter offers protein, healthy fats, and additional nutrients.

Preparation Time: 3 minutes

8. Chickpea Salad Lettuce Wraps

Ingredients:

> ➤ 1 cup cooked chickpeas

> ➤ 1/4 cup diced bell peppers

> ➤ 1/4 cup diced cucumber

> ➤ 1/4 cup diced tomatoes

- ➤ 1 tablespoon chopped fresh parsley or cilantro
- ➤ 1 tablespoon lemon juice
- ➤ Salt and pepper to taste
- ➤ Lettuce leaves for wrapping

Instructions:

- ➤ In a mixing bowl, combine cooked chickpeas, diced bell peppers, cucumber, tomatoes, parsley or cilantro, lemon juice, salt, and pepper.
- ➤ Mix until well combined.
- ➤ Spoon the chickpea salad onto lettuce leaves.
- ➤ Roll up the lettuce leaves to form wraps.
- ➤ Serve immediately.

Health Benefits:

- ➤ Chickpeas are a good source of plant-based protein and fiber, while vegetables provide vitamins, minerals, and antioxidants.
- ➤ Lettuce leaves offer a low-calorie base for the wraps.

Preparation Time: 10 minutes

9. Edamame

Ingredients:

- ➢ 1 cup frozen edamame (in pods)
- ➢ Salt to taste

Instructions:

- ➢ Bring a pot of water to a boil.
- ➢ Add frozen edamame to the boiling water and cook for 3-5 minutes, or until tender.
- ➢ Drain the edamame and rinse with cold water.
- ➢ Sprinkle with salt to taste.
- ➢ Serve chilled or at room temperature.

Health Benefits:

- ➢ Edamame is rich in plant-based protein, fiber, vitamins, and minerals like folate and manganese, supporting muscle repair, satiety, and overall health.

Preparation Time: 10 minutes

10. Roasted Chickpeas

Ingredients:

- ➢ 1 can (15 ounces) chickpeas, drained and rinsed

- ➢ 1 tablespoon olive oil
- ➢ 1 teaspoon ground cumin
- ➢ 1/2 teaspoon paprika
- ➢ 1/2 teaspoon garlic powder
- ➢ Salt to taste

Instructions:

- ➢ Preheat the oven to 400°F (200°C).
- ➢ Pat the chickpeas dry with a clean kitchen towel or paper towels.
- ➢ In a bowl, toss the chickpeas with olive oil, ground cumin, paprika, garlic powder, and salt until evenly coated.
- ➢ Spread the seasoned chickpeas in a single layer on a baking sheet lined with parchment paper.
- ➢ Roast in the preheated oven for 25-30 minutes, or until golden brown and crispy, shaking the pan halfway through cooking.
- ➢ Remove from the oven and let cool before serving.

Health Benefits:

> ➤ Roasted chickpeas are a crunchy and satisfying snack, providing plant-based protein, fiber, and essential nutrients like iron and magnesium.

Preparation Time: 35 minutes

CONCLUSION

Embarking on a plant-based weight loss journey offers not only a path to achieving your desired weight but also a transformative approach to nourishing your body, sustaining your health, and embracing a more compassionate lifestyle.

This cookbook serves as a comprehensive guide, providing a diverse array of delicious and nutritious recipes meticulously crafted to support your weight loss goals while tantalizing your taste buds.

Through the power of whole, plant-derived foods, you'll discover a newfound appreciation for the abundance of flavors, textures, and nutrients nature has to offer.

From vibrant salads bursting with color to hearty stews brimming with wholesome goodness, each recipe invites you to explore the endless possibilities of plant-based cuisine.

But beyond the culinary delights, this cookbook is a testament to the profound impact that conscious eating can have on our bodies, our communities, and our planet.

By choosing plant-based foods, you're not just nourishing yourself; you're contributing to a more sustainable and compassionate world.

As you embark on this journey, remember that sustainable weight loss is not about restriction or deprivation but rather about embracing abundance, balance, and mindfulness in your eating habits.

So savor each bite, listen to your body's cues, and celebrate the joy of nourishing yourself from the inside out.

May this cookbook be your trusted companion on your plant-based weight loss journey, guiding you towards a healthier, happier, and more vibrant life.

Here's to good health, good food, and the power of plants to transform our lives for the better.